CALORIE COUNTER
JOURNAL & LOGBOOK

CALORIE COUNTER JOURNAL & LOGBOOK

KEEP TRACK OF YOUR DAILY CALORIES,
EXERCISE, WEEKLY STATS & GOALS
WITH SPACE FOR JOURNAL ENTRIES & NOTES

KIMBERLY EDDLEMAN

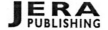
JERA
PUBLISHING

AN IMPRINT OF JERA WEB CREATIONS, LLC
GEORGIA, USA

CALORIE COUNTER JOURNAL & LOGBOOK

Copyright © 2006 by Kimberly Ann Eddleman

ISBN 0-9768076-5-3

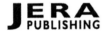

Published by Jera Publishing
an imprint of Jera Web Creations, LLC
http://www.jerapublishing.com

Printed in the United States of America

MEAL ITEMS

Use the following pages to write down your common meal items along with their serving size and calories. This will make it easier to log your daily meals in the main section since you have already calculated the calories.

Combine all ingredients into one meal item list. For instance, the listing for a spaghetti dinner with meat sauce should include the combined calories of the pasta, sauce, meat and anything else usually added to it.

When writing down the serving size for the meal use something that is meaningful and easy for you to you to follow and not necessarily the serving size on the package. Using "4 oz" as a serving size for that spaghetti dinner isn't very helpful but "1 small bowl" will be easier to understand.

When adding to your daily log you can then just enter "Spaghetti Dinner" along with its calories that you have already calculated. If you have more than one of your normal serving just enter "Spaghetti Dinner x 2" and double the calories.

BREAKFAST

MEAL ITEM	SERVING	CALORIES	FROM FAT

BREAKFAST

MEAL ITEM	SERVING	CALORIES	FROM FAT

LUNCH

MEAL ITEM	SERVING	CALORIES	FROM FAT

LUNCH

MEAL ITEM	SERVING	CALORIES	FROM FAT

DINNER

MEAL ITEM	SERVING	CALORIES	FROM FAT

DINNER

MEAL ITEM	SERVING	CALORIES	FROM FAT

SIDE DISHES

MEAL ITEM	SERVING	CALORIES	FROM FAT

SNACKS/BEVERAGES

MEAL ITEM	SERVING	CALORIES	FROM FAT

JOURNAL & LOGBOOK

Each week will start with an area to record your weekly stats such as weight and body measurements to help track your progress. Blank spaces are included to record a stat not listed.

The week is divided into daily pages with tables for breakfast, lunch, dinner and snacks. Write down caloric intake goal for the day, your meals and the calories consumed for each meal. A column for tracking calories from fat is also provided as well as calories burned from exercise.

At the end of the day total up your total calories consumed, calories from fat, calories burned and the adjusted calories (total minus burned).

Places to jot down notes or journal entries are available at the start of each week, the end of each day, the end of every week and the last pages of the logbook.

WEEK ONE

STARTING STATS

DATE:	WEIGHT:
WAIST:	HIPS:
CHEST:	THIGHS:
CALVES:	ARMS:

NOTES/JOURNAL/GOALS

_____

_____

_____

_____

_____

_____

_____

_____

_____

_____

_____

_____

_____

SUNDAY:

CALORIC INTAKE GOAL

BREAKFAST	CALORIES	FROM FAT
MEAL TOTAL:		

LUNCH	CALORIES	FROM FAT
MEAL TOTAL:		

DINNER	CALORIES	FROM FAT
MEAL TOTAL:		

SNACKS/DESSERTS	CALORIES	FROM FAT
TOTAL:		

EXERCISE	CALORIES BURNED
TOTAL CALORIES BURNED:	

CALORIE TOTALS

INTAKE	FROM FAT	BURNED	ADJUSTED

NOTES

MONDAY:

CALORIC INTAKE GOAL

BREAKFAST	CALORIES	FROM FAT
MEAL TOTAL:		

LUNCH	CALORIES	FROM FAT
MEAL TOTAL:		

DINNER	CALORIES	FROM FAT
MEAL TOTAL:		

SNACKS/DESSERTS	CALORIES	FROM FAT
TOTAL:		

EXERCISE	CALORIES BURNED
TOTAL CALORIES BURNED:	

CALORIE TOTALS

INTAKE	FROM FAT	BURNED	ADJUSTED

NOTES

TUESDAY:

CALORIC INTAKE GOAL

BREAKFAST	CALORIES	FROM FAT
MEAL TOTAL:		

LUNCH	CALORIES	FROM FAT
MEAL TOTAL:		

DINNER	CALORIES	FROM FAT
MEAL TOTAL:		

6

SNACKS/DESSERTS	CALORIES	FROM FAT
TOTAL:		

EXERCISE	CALORIES BURNED
TOTAL CALORIES BURNED:	

CALORIE TOTALS

INTAKE	FROM FAT	BURNED	ADJUSTED

NOTES

WEDNESDAY:

CALORIC INTAKE GOAL

BREAKFAST	CALORIES	FROM FAT
MEAL TOTAL:		

LUNCH	CALORIES	FROM FAT
MEAL TOTAL:		

DINNER	CALORIES	FROM FAT
MEAL TOTAL:		

SNACKS/DESSERTS	CALORIES	FROM FAT
TOTAL:		

EXERCISE	CALORIES BURNED
TOTAL CALORIES BURNED:	

CALORIE TOTALS

INTAKE	FROM FAT	BURNED	ADJUSTED

NOTES

THURSDAY:

CALORIC INTAKE GOAL

BREAKFAST	CALORIES	FROM FAT
MEAL TOTAL:		

LUNCH	CALORIES	FROM FAT
MEAL TOTAL:		

DINNER	CALORIES	FROM FAT
MEAL TOTAL:		

SNACKS/DESSERTS	CALORIES	FROM FAT
TOTAL:		

EXERCISE	CALORIES BURNED
TOTAL CALORIES BURNED:	

CALORIE TOTALS

INTAKE	FROM FAT	BURNED	ADJUSTED

NOTES

FRIDAY:

CALORIC INTAKE GOAL

BREAKFAST	CALORIES	FROM FAT
MEAL TOTAL:		

LUNCH	CALORIES	FROM FAT
MEAL TOTAL:		

DINNER	CALORIES	FROM FAT
MEAL TOTAL:		

SNACKS/DESSERTS	CALORIES	FROM FAT
TOTAL:		

EXERCISE	CALORIES BURNED
TOTAL CALORIES BURNED:	

CALORIE TOTALS

INTAKE	FROM FAT	BURNED	ADJUSTED

NOTES

13

SATURDAY:

CALORIC INTAKE GOAL

BREAKFAST	CALORIES	FROM FAT
MEAL TOTAL:		

LUNCH	CALORIES	FROM FAT
MEAL TOTAL:		

DINNER	CALORIES	FROM FAT
MEAL TOTAL:		

SNACKS/DESSERTS	CALORIES	FROM FAT
TOTAL:		

EXERCISE	CALORIES BURNED
TOTAL CALORIES BURNED:	

CALORIE TOTALS

INTAKE	FROM FAT	BURNED	ADJUSTED

NOTES

_____

_____

_____

_____

_____

END OF WEEK ONE NOTES/JOURNAL

WEEK TWO

STARTING STATS

DATE:	WEIGHT:
WAIST:	HIPS:
CHEST:	THIGHS:
CALVES:	ARMS:

NOTES/JOURNAL/GOALS

_____

_____

_____

_____

_____

_____

_____

_____

_____

_____

_____

_____

_____

SUNDAY:

CALORIC INTAKE GOAL

BREAKFAST	CALORIES	FROM FAT
MEAL TOTAL:		

LUNCH	CALORIES	FROM FAT
MEAL TOTAL:		

DINNER	CALORIES	FROM FAT
MEAL TOTAL:		

SNACKS/DESSERTS	CALORIES	FROM FAT
TOTAL:		

EXERCISE	CALORIES BURNED
TOTAL CALORIES BURNED:	

CALORIE TOTALS

INTAKE	FROM FAT	BURNED	ADJUSTED

NOTES

MONDAY:

CALORIC INTAKE GOAL

BREAKFAST	CALORIES	FROM FAT
MEAL TOTAL:		

LUNCH	CALORIES	FROM FAT
MEAL TOTAL:		

DINNER	CALORIES	FROM FAT
MEAL TOTAL:		

SNACKS/DESSERTS	CALORIES	FROM FAT
TOTAL:		

EXERCISE	CALORIES BURNED
TOTAL CALORIES BURNED:	

CALORIE TOTALS

INTAKE	FROM FAT	BURNED	ADJUSTED

NOTES

TUESDAY:

CALORIC INTAKE GOAL

BREAKFAST	CALORIES	FROM FAT
MEAL TOTAL:		

LUNCH	CALORIES	FROM FAT
MEAL TOTAL:		

DINNER	CALORIES	FROM FAT
MEAL TOTAL:		

SNACKS/DESSERTS	CALORIES	FROM FAT
TOTAL:		

EXERCISE	CALORIES BURNED
TOTAL CALORIES BURNED:	

CALORIE TOTALS

INTAKE	FROM FAT	BURNED	ADJUSTED

NOTES

23

WEDNESDAY:

CALORIC INTAKE GOAL

BREAKFAST	CALORIES	FROM FAT
MEAL TOTAL:		

LUNCH	CALORIES	FROM FAT
MEAL TOTAL:		

DINNER	CALORIES	FROM FAT
MEAL TOTAL:		

SNACKS/DESSERTS	CALORIES	FROM FAT
TOTAL:		

EXERCISE	CALORIES BURNED
TOTAL CALORIES BURNED:	

CALORIE TOTALS

INTAKE	FROM FAT	BURNED	ADJUSTED

NOTES

_____

_____

_____

_____

THURSDAY:

CALORIC INTAKE GOAL

BREAKFAST	CALORIES	FROM FAT
MEAL TOTAL:		

LUNCH	CALORIES	FROM FAT
MEAL TOTAL:		

DINNER	CALORIES	FROM FAT
MEAL TOTAL:		

26

SNACKS/DESSERTS	CALORIES	FROM FAT
TOTAL:		

EXERCISE	CALORIES BURNED
TOTAL CALORIES BURNED:	

CALORIE TOTALS

INTAKE	FROM FAT	BURNED	ADJUSTED

NOTES

FRIDAY:

CALORIC INTAKE GOAL

BREAKFAST	CALORIES	FROM FAT
MEAL TOTAL:		

LUNCH	CALORIES	FROM FAT
MEAL TOTAL:		

DINNER	CALORIES	FROM FAT
MEAL TOTAL:		

SNACKS/DESSERTS	CALORIES	FROM FAT
TOTAL:		

EXERCISE	CALORIES BURNED
TOTAL CALORIES BURNED:	

CALORIE TOTALS

INTAKE	FROM FAT	BURNED	ADJUSTED

NOTES

SATURDAY:

CALORIC INTAKE GOAL

BREAKFAST	CALORIES	FROM FAT
MEAL TOTAL:		

LUNCH	CALORIES	FROM FAT
MEAL TOTAL:		

DINNER	CALORIES	FROM FAT
MEAL TOTAL:		

SNACKS/DESSERTS	CALORIES	FROM FAT
TOTAL:		

EXERCISE	CALORIES BURNED
TOTAL CALORIES BURNED:	

CALORIE TOTALS

INTAKE	FROM FAT	BURNED	ADJUSTED

NOTES

WEEK THREE

STARTING STATS

DATE:	WEIGHT:
WAIST:	HIPS:
CHEST:	THIGHS:
CALVES:	ARMS:

NOTES/JOURNAL/GOALS

SUNDAY:

CALORIC INTAKE GOAL

BREAKFAST	CALORIES	FROM FAT
MEAL TOTAL:		

LUNCH	CALORIES	FROM FAT
MEAL TOTAL:		

DINNER	CALORIES	FROM FAT
MEAL TOTAL:		

SNACKS/DESSERTS	CALORIES	FROM FAT
TOTAL:		

EXERCISE	CALORIES BURNED
TOTAL CALORIES BURNED:	

CALORIE TOTALS

INTAKE	FROM FAT	BURNED	ADJUSTED

NOTES

MONDAY:

CALORIC INTAKE GOAL

BREAKFAST	CALORIES	FROM FAT
MEAL TOTAL:		

LUNCH	CALORIES	FROM FAT
MEAL TOTAL:		

DINNER	CALORIES	FROM FAT
MEAL TOTAL:		

SNACKS/DESSERTS	CALORIES	FROM FAT
TOTAL:		

EXERCISE	CALORIES BURNED
TOTAL CALORIES BURNED:	

CALORIE TOTALS

INTAKE	FROM FAT	BURNED	ADJUSTED

NOTES

_____

_____

_____

_____

TUESDAY:

CALORIC INTAKE GOAL

BREAKFAST	CALORIES	FROM FAT
MEAL TOTAL:		

LUNCH	CALORIES	FROM FAT
MEAL TOTAL:		

DINNER	CALORIES	FROM FAT
MEAL TOTAL:		

SNACKS/DESSERTS

SNACKS/DESSERTS	CALORIES	FROM FAT
TOTAL:		

EXERCISE

EXERCISE	CALORIES BURNED
TOTAL CALORIES BURNED:	

CALORIE TOTALS

INTAKE	FROM FAT	BURNED	ADJUSTED

NOTES

WEDNESDAY:

CALORIC INTAKE GOAL

BREAKFAST	CALORIES	FROM FAT
MEAL TOTAL:		

LUNCH	CALORIES	FROM FAT
MEAL TOTAL:		

DINNER	CALORIES	FROM FAT
MEAL TOTAL:		

SNACKS/DESSERTS	CALORIES	FROM FAT
TOTAL:		

EXERCISE	CALORIES BURNED
TOTAL CALORIES BURNED:	

CALORIE TOTALS

INTAKE	FROM FAT	BURNED	ADJUSTED

NOTES

THURSDAY:

CALORIC INTAKE GOAL

BREAKFAST	CALORIES	FROM FAT
MEAL TOTAL:		

LUNCH	CALORIES	FROM FAT
MEAL TOTAL:		

DINNER	CALORIES	FROM FAT
MEAL TOTAL:		

SNACKS/DESSERTS	CALORIES	FROM FAT
TOTAL:		

EXERCISE	CALORIES BURNED
TOTAL CALORIES BURNED:	

CALORIE TOTALS

INTAKE	FROM FAT	BURNED	ADJUSTED

NOTES

FRIDAY:

CALORIC INTAKE GOAL

BREAKFAST	CALORIES	FROM FAT
MEAL TOTAL:		

LUNCH	CALORIES	FROM FAT
MEAL TOTAL:		

DINNER	CALORIES	FROM FAT
MEAL TOTAL:		

SNACKS/DESSERTS	CALORIES	FROM FAT
TOTAL:		

EXERCISE	CALORIES BURNED
TOTAL CALORIES BURNED:	

CALORIE TOTALS

INTAKE	FROM FAT	BURNED	ADJUSTED

NOTES

SATURDAY:

CALORIC INTAKE GOAL

BREAKFAST	CALORIES	FROM FAT
MEAL TOTAL:		

LUNCH	CALORIES	FROM FAT
MEAL TOTAL:		

DINNER	CALORIES	FROM FAT
MEAL TOTAL:		

SNACKS/DESSERTS	CALORIES	FROM FAT
TOTAL:		

EXERCISE	CALORIES BURNED
TOTAL CALORIES BURNED:	

CALORIE TOTALS

INTAKE	FROM FAT	BURNED	ADJUSTED

NOTES

47

WEEK FOUR

STARTING STATS

DATE:	WEIGHT:
WAIST:	HIPS:
CHEST:	THIGHS:
CALVES:	ARMS:

NOTES/JOURNAL/GOALS

_____

_____

_____

_____

_____

_____

_____

_____

_____

_____

_____

_____

_____

SUNDAY:

CALORIC INTAKE GOAL

BREAKFAST	CALORIES	FROM FAT
MEAL TOTAL:		

LUNCH	CALORIES	FROM FAT
MEAL TOTAL:		

DINNER	CALORIES	FROM FAT
MEAL TOTAL:		

50

SNACKS/DESSERTS	CALORIES	FROM FAT
TOTAL:		

EXERCISE	CALORIES BURNED
TOTAL CALORIES BURNED:	

CALORIE TOTALS

INTAKE	FROM FAT	BURNED	ADJUSTED

NOTES

MONDAY:

CALORIC INTAKE GOAL

BREAKFAST	CALORIES	FROM FAT
MEAL TOTAL:		

LUNCH	CALORIES	FROM FAT
MEAL TOTAL:		

DINNER	CALORIES	FROM FAT
MEAL TOTAL:		

SNACKS/DESSERTS	CALORIES	FROM FAT
TOTAL:		

EXERCISE	CALORIES BURNED
TOTAL CALORIES BURNED:	

CALORIE TOTALS

INTAKE	FROM FAT	BURNED	ADJUSTED

NOTES

TUESDAY:

CALORIC INTAKE GOAL

BREAKFAST	CALORIES	FROM FAT
MEAL TOTAL:		

LUNCH	CALORIES	FROM FAT
MEAL TOTAL:		

DINNER	CALORIES	FROM FAT
MEAL TOTAL:		

54

SNACKS/DESSERTS

	CALORIES	FROM FAT
TOTAL:		

EXERCISE

	CALORIES BURNED
TOTAL CALORIES BURNED:	

CALORIE TOTALS

INTAKE	FROM FAT	BURNED	ADJUSTED

NOTES

WEDNESDAY:

CALORIC INTAKE GOAL

BREAKFAST	CALORIES	FROM FAT
MEAL TOTAL:		

LUNCH	CALORIES	FROM FAT
MEAL TOTAL:		

DINNER	CALORIES	FROM FAT
MEAL TOTAL:		

SNACKS/DESSERTS	CALORIES	FROM FAT
TOTAL:		

EXERCISE	CALORIES BURNED
TOTAL CALORIES BURNED:	

CALORIE TOTALS

INTAKE	FROM FAT	BURNED	ADJUSTED

NOTES

SDAY:

CALORIC INTAKE GOAL

BREAKFAST	CALORIES	FROM FAT
MEAL TOTAL:		

LUNCH	CALORIES	FROM FAT
MEAL TOTAL:		

DINNER	CALORIES	FROM FAT
MEAL TOTAL:		

SNACKS/DESSERTS	CALORIES	FROM FAT
TOTAL:		

EXERCISE	CALORIES BURNED
TOTAL CALORIES BURNED:	

CALORIE TOTALS

INTAKE	FROM FAT	BURNED	ADJUSTED

NOTES

FRIDAY:

CALORIC INTAKE GOAL

BREAKFAST	CALORIES	FROM FAT
MEAL TOTAL:		

LUNCH	CALORIES	FROM FAT
MEAL TOTAL:		

DINNER	CALORIES	FROM FAT
MEAL TOTAL:		

SNACKS/DESSERTS	CALORIES	FROM FAT
TOTAL:		

EXERCISE	CALORIES BURNED
TOTAL CALORIES BURNED:	

CALORIE TOTALS

INTAKE	FROM FAT	BURNED	ADJUSTED

NOTES

61

SATURDAY:

CALORIC INTAKE GOAL

BREAKFAST	CALORIES	FROM FAT
MEAL TOTAL:		

LUNCH	CALORIES	FROM FAT
MEAL TOTAL:		

DINNER	CALORIES	FROM FAT
MEAL TOTAL:		

SNACKS/DESSERTS	CALORIES	FROM FAT
TOTAL:		

EXERCISE	CALORIES BURNED
TOTAL CALORIES BURNED:	

CALORIE TOTALS

INTAKE	FROM FAT	BURNED	ADJUSTED

NOTES

_____

_____

_____

_____

WEEK FIVE

STARTING STATS

DATE:	WEIGHT:
WAIST:	HIPS:
CHEST:	THIGHS:
CALVES:	ARMS:

NOTES/JOURNAL/GOALS

_____

_____

_____

_____

_____

_____

_____

_____

_____

_____

_____

SUNDAY:

CALORIC INTAKE GOAL

BREAKFAST	CALORIES	FROM FAT
MEAL TOTAL:		

LUNCH	CALORIES	FROM FAT
MEAL TOTAL:		

DINNER	CALORIES	FROM FAT
MEAL TOTAL:		

SNACKS/DESSERTS	CALORIES	FROM FAT
TOTAL:		

EXERCISE	CALORIES BURNED
TOTAL CALORIES BURNED:	

CALORIE TOTALS

INTAKE	FROM FAT	BURNED	ADJUSTED

NOTES

MONDAY:

CALORIC INTAKE GOAL

BREAKFAST	CALORIES	FROM FAT
MEAL TOTAL:		

LUNCH	CALORIES	FROM FAT
MEAL TOTAL:		

DINNER	CALORIES	FROM FAT
MEAL TOTAL:		

SNACKS/DESSERTS	CALORIES	FROM FAT
TOTAL:		

EXERCISE	CALORIES BURNED
TOTAL CALORIES BURNED:	

CALORIE TOTALS

INTAKE	FROM FAT	BURNED	ADJUSTED

NOTES

TUESDAY:

CALORIC INTAKE GOAL

BREAKFAST	CALORIES	FROM FAT
MEAL TOTAL:		

LUNCH	CALORIES	FROM FAT
MEAL TOTAL:		

DINNER	CALORIES	FROM FAT
MEAL TOTAL:		

70

SNACKS/DESSERTS	CALORIES	FROM FAT
TOTAL:		

EXERCISE	CALORIES BURNED
TOTAL CALORIES BURNED:	

CALORIE TOTALS

INTAKE	FROM FAT	BURNED	ADJUSTED

NOTES

WEDNESDAY:

CALORIC INTAKE GOAL

BREAKFAST	CALORIES	FROM FAT
MEAL TOTAL:		

LUNCH	CALORIES	FROM FAT
MEAL TOTAL:		

DINNER	CALORIES	FROM FAT
MEAL TOTAL:		

SNACKS/DESSERTS	CALORIES	FROM FAT
TOTAL:		

EXERCISE	CALORIES BURNED
TOTAL CALORIES BURNED:	

CALORIE TOTALS

INTAKE	FROM FAT	BURNED	ADJUSTED

NOTES

THURSDAY:

CALORIC INTAKE GOAL

BREAKFAST	CALORIES	FROM FAT
MEAL TOTAL:		

LUNCH	CALORIES	FROM FAT
MEAL TOTAL:		

DINNER	CALORIES	FROM FAT
MEAL TOTAL:		

74

SNACKS/DESSERTS	CALORIES	FROM FAT
TOTAL:		

EXERCISE	CALORIES BURNED
TOTAL CALORIES BURNED:	

CALORIE TOTALS

INTAKE	FROM FAT	BURNED	ADJUSTED

NOTES

FRIDAY:

CALORIC INTAKE GOAL

BREAKFAST	CALORIES	FROM FAT
MEAL TOTAL:		

LUNCH	CALORIES	FROM FAT
MEAL TOTAL:		

DINNER	CALORIES	FROM FAT
MEAL TOTAL:		

SNACKS/DESSERTS	CALORIES	FROM FAT
TOTAL:		

EXERCISE	CALORIES BURNED
TOTAL CALORIES BURNED:	

CALORIE TOTALS

INTAKE	FROM FAT	BURNED	ADJUSTED

NOTES

SATURDAY:

CALORIC INTAKE GOAL

BREAKFAST	CALORIES	FROM FAT
MEAL TOTAL:		

LUNCH	CALORIES	FROM FAT
MEAL TOTAL:		

DINNER	CALORIES	FROM FAT
MEAL TOTAL:		

SNACKS/DESSERTS	CALORIES	FROM FAT
TOTAL:		

EXERCISE	CALORIES BURNED
TOTAL CALORIES BURNED:	

CALORIE TOTALS

INTAKE	FROM FAT	BURNED	ADJUSTED

NOTES

WEEK SIX

STARTING STATS

DATE:	WEIGHT:
WAIST:	HIPS:
CHEST:	THIGHS:
CALVES:	ARMS:

NOTES/JOURNAL/GOALS

_____

_____

_____

_____

_____

_____

_____

_____

_____

_____

_____

_____

_____

SUNDAY:

CALORIC INTAKE GOAL

BREAKFAST	CALORIES	FROM FAT
MEAL TOTAL:		

LUNCH	CALORIES	FROM FAT
MEAL TOTAL:		

DINNER	CALORIES	FROM FAT
MEAL TOTAL:		

SNACKS/DESSERTS	CALORIES	FROM FAT
TOTAL:		

EXERCISE	CALORIES BURNED
TOTAL CALORIES BURNED:	

CALORIE TOTALS

INTAKE	FROM FAT	BURNED	ADJUSTED

NOTES

MONDAY:

CALORIC INTAKE GOAL

BREAKFAST	CALORIES	FROM FAT
MEAL TOTAL:		

LUNCH	CALORIES	FROM FAT
MEAL TOTAL:		

DINNER	CALORIES	FROM FAT
MEAL TOTAL:		

SNACKS/DESSERTS	CALORIES	FROM FAT
TOTAL:		

EXERCISE	CALORIES BURNED
TOTAL CALORIES BURNED:	

CALORIE TOTALS

INTAKE	FROM FAT	BURNED	ADJUSTED

NOTES

TUESDAY:

CALORIC INTAKE GOAL

BREAKFAST	CALORIES	FROM FAT
MEAL TOTAL:		

LUNCH	CALORIES	FROM FAT
MEAL TOTAL:		

DINNER	CALORIES	FROM FAT
MEAL TOTAL:		

SNACKS/DESSERTS	CALORIES	FROM FAT
TOTAL:		

EXERCISE	CALORIES BURNED
TOTAL CALORIES BURNED:	

CALORIE TOTALS

INTAKE	FROM FAT	BURNED	ADJUSTED

NOTES

WEDNESDAY:

CALORIC INTAKE GOAL

BREAKFAST

	CALORIES	FROM FAT
MEAL TOTAL:		

LUNCH

	CALORIES	FROM FAT
MEAL TOTAL:		

DINNER

	CALORIES	FROM FAT
MEAL TOTAL:		

SNACKS/DESSERTS

	CALORIES	FROM FAT
TOTAL:		

EXERCISE

	CALORIES BURNED
TOTAL CALORIES BURNED:	

CALORIE TOTALS

INTAKE	FROM FAT	BURNED	ADJUSTED

NOTES

THURSDAY:

CALORIC INTAKE GOAL

BREAKFAST	CALORIES	FROM FAT
MEAL TOTAL:		

LUNCH	CALORIES	FROM FAT
MEAL TOTAL:		

DINNER	CALORIES	FROM FAT
MEAL TOTAL:		

SNACKS/DESSERTS	CALORIES	FROM FAT
TOTAL:		

EXERCISE	CALORIES BURNED
TOTAL CALORIES BURNED:	

CALORIE TOTALS

INTAKE	FROM FAT	BURNED	ADJUSTED

NOTES

FRIDAY:

CALORIC INTAKE GOAL

BREAKFAST	CALORIES	FROM FAT
MEAL TOTAL:		

LUNCH	CALORIES	FROM FAT
MEAL TOTAL:		

DINNER	CALORIES	FROM FAT
MEAL TOTAL:		

SNACKS/DESSERTS	CALORIES	FROM FAT
TOTAL:		

EXERCISE	CALORIES BURNED
TOTAL CALORIES BURNED:	

CALORIE TOTALS

INTAKE	FROM FAT	BURNED	ADJUSTED

NOTES

93

SATURDAY:

CALORIC INTAKE GOAL

BREAKFAST	CALORIES	FROM FAT
MEAL TOTAL:		

LUNCH	CALORIES	FROM FAT
MEAL TOTAL:		

DINNER	CALORIES	FROM FAT
MEAL TOTAL:		

SNACKS/DESSERTS	CALORIES	FROM FAT
TOTAL:		

EXERCISE	CALORIES BURNED
TOTAL CALORIES BURNED:	

CALORIE TOTALS

INTAKE	FROM FAT	BURNED	ADJUSTED

NOTES

WEEK SEVEN

STARTING STATS

DATE:	WEIGHT:
WAIST:	HIPS:
CHEST:	THIGHS:
CALVES:	ARMS:

NOTES/JOURNAL/GOALS

_____

_____

_____

_____

_____

_____

_____

_____

_____

_____

_____

_____

_____

SUNDAY:

CALORIC INTAKE GOAL

BREAKFAST	CALORIES	FROM FAT
MEAL TOTAL:		

LUNCH	CALORIES	FROM FAT
MEAL TOTAL:		

DINNER	CALORIES	FROM FAT
MEAL TOTAL:		

SNACKS/DESSERTS	CALORIES	FROM FAT
TOTAL:		

EXERCISE	CALORIES BURNED
TOTAL CALORIES BURNED:	

CALORIE TOTALS

INTAKE	FROM FAT	BURNED	ADJUSTED

NOTES

MONDAY:

CALORIC INTAKE GOAL

BREAKFAST	CALORIES	FROM FAT
MEAL TOTAL:		

LUNCH	CALORIES	FROM FAT
MEAL TOTAL:		

DINNER	CALORIES	FROM FAT
MEAL TOTAL:		

SNACKS/DESSERTS	CALORIES	FROM FAT
TOTAL:		

EXERCISE	CALORIES BURNED
TOTAL CALORIES BURNED:	

CALORIE TOTALS

INTAKE	FROM FAT	BURNED	ADJUSTED

NOTES

TUESDAY:

CALORIC INTAKE GOAL

BREAKFAST	CALORIES	FROM FAT
MEAL TOTAL:		

LUNCH	CALORIES	FROM FAT
MEAL TOTAL:		

DINNER	CALORIES	FROM FAT
MEAL TOTAL:		

SNACKS/DESSERTS	CALORIES	FROM FAT
TOTAL:		

EXERCISE	CALORIES BURNED
TOTAL CALORIES BURNED:	

CALORIE TOTALS

INTAKE	FROM FAT	BURNED	ADJUSTED

NOTES

WEDNESDAY:

CALORIC INTAKE GOAL

BREAKFAST	CALORIES	FROM FAT
MEAL TOTAL:		

LUNCH	CALORIES	FROM FAT
MEAL TOTAL:		

DINNER	CALORIES	FROM FAT
MEAL TOTAL:		

SNACKS/DESSERTS	CALORIES	FROM FAT
TOTAL:		

EXERCISE	CALORIES BURNED
TOTAL CALORIES BURNED:	

CALORIE TOTALS

INTAKE	FROM FAT	BURNED	ADJUSTED

NOTES

THURSDAY:

CALORIC INTAKE GOAL

BREAKFAST	CALORIES	FROM FAT
MEAL TOTAL:		

LUNCH	CALORIES	FROM FAT
MEAL TOTAL:		

DINNER	CALORIES	FROM FAT
MEAL TOTAL:		

SNACKS/DESSERTS	CALORIES	FROM FAT
TOTAL:		

EXERCISE	CALORIES BURNED
TOTAL CALORIES BURNED:	

CALORIE TOTALS

INTAKE	FROM FAT	BURNED	ADJUSTED

NOTES

FRIDAY:

CALORIC INTAKE GOAL

BREAKFAST	CALORIES	FROM FAT
MEAL TOTAL:		

LUNCH	CALORIES	FROM FAT
MEAL TOTAL:		

DINNER	CALORIES	FROM FAT
MEAL TOTAL:		

SNACKS/DESSERTS	CALORIES	FROM FAT
TOTAL:		

EXERCISE	CALORIES BURNED
TOTAL CALORIES BURNED:	

CALORIE TOTALS

INTAKE	FROM FAT	BURNED	ADJUSTED

NOTES

SATURDAY:

CALORIC INTAKE GOAL

BREAKFAST	CALORIES	FROM FAT
MEAL TOTAL:		

LUNCH	CALORIES	FROM FAT
MEAL TOTAL:		

DINNER	CALORIES	FROM FAT
MEAL TOTAL:		

SNACKS/DESSERTS	CALORIES	FROM FAT
TOTAL:		

EXERCISE	CALORIES BURNED
TOTAL CALORIES BURNED:	

CALORIE TOTALS

INTAKE	FROM FAT	BURNED	ADJUSTED

NOTES

111

WEEK EIGHT

STARTING STATS

DATE:	WEIGHT:
WAIST:	HIPS:
CHEST:	THIGHS:
CALVES:	ARMS:

NOTES/JOURNAL/GOALS

_____

_____

_____

_____

_____

_____

_____

_____

_____

_____

_____

_____

_____

SUNDAY:

CALORIC INTAKE GOAL

BREAKFAST	CALORIES	FROM FAT
MEAL TOTAL:		

LUNCH	CALORIES	FROM FAT
MEAL TOTAL:		

DINNER	CALORIES	FROM FAT
MEAL TOTAL:		

SNACKS/DESSERTS	CALORIES	FROM FAT
TOTAL:		

EXERCISE	CALORIES BURNED
TOTAL CALORIES BURNED:	

CALORIE TOTALS

INTAKE	FROM FAT	BURNED	ADJUSTED

NOTES

115

MONDAY:

CALORIC INTAKE GOAL

BREAKFAST

	CALORIES	FROM FAT
MEAL TOTAL:		

LUNCH

	CALORIES	FROM FAT
MEAL TOTAL:		

DINNER

	CALORIES	FROM FAT
MEAL TOTAL:		

SNACKS/DESSERTS	CALORIES	FROM FAT
TOTAL:		

EXERCISE	CALORIES BURNED
TOTAL CALORIES BURNED:	

CALORIE TOTALS

INTAKE	FROM FAT	BURNED	ADJUSTED

NOTES

117

TUESDAY:

CALORIC INTAKE GOAL

BREAKFAST	CALORIES	FROM FAT
MEAL TOTAL:		

LUNCH	CALORIES	FROM FAT
MEAL TOTAL:		

DINNER	CALORIES	FROM FAT
MEAL TOTAL:		

SNACKS/DESSERTS	CALORIES	FROM FAT
TOTAL:		

EXERCISE	CALORIES BURNED
TOTAL CALORIES BURNED:	

CALORIE TOTALS

INTAKE	FROM FAT	BURNED	ADJUSTED

NOTES

WEDNESDAY:

BREAKFAST

	CALORIES	FROM FAT
MEAL TOTAL:		

LUNCH

	CALORIES	FROM FAT
MEAL TOTAL:		

DINNER

	CALORIES	FROM FAT
MEAL TOTAL:		

SNACKS/DESSERTS	CALORIES	FROM FAT
TOTAL:		

EXERCISE	CALORIES BURNED
TOTAL CALORIES BURNED:	

CALORIE TOTALS

INTAKE	FROM FAT	BURNED	ADJUSTED

NOTES

THURSDAY:

CALORIC INTAKE GOAL

BREAKFAST	CALORIES	FROM FAT
MEAL TOTAL:		

LUNCH	CALORIES	FROM FAT
MEAL TOTAL:		

DINNER	CALORIES	FROM FAT
MEAL TOTAL:		

SNACKS/DESSERTS	CALORIES	FROM FAT
TOTAL:		

EXERCISE	CALORIES BURNED
TOTAL CALORIES BURNED:	

CALORIE TOTALS

INTAKE	FROM FAT	BURNED	ADJUSTED

NOTES

FRIDAY:

CALORIC INTAKE GOAL

BREAKFAST	CALORIES	FROM FAT
MEAL TOTAL:		

LUNCH	CALORIES	FROM FAT
MEAL TOTAL:		

DINNER	CALORIES	FROM FAT
MEAL TOTAL:		

124

SNACKS/DESSERTS	CALORIES	FROM FAT
TOTAL:		

EXERCISE	CALORIES BURNED
TOTAL CALORIES BURNED:	

CALORIE TOTALS

INTAKE	FROM FAT	BURNED	ADJUSTED

NOTES

SATURDAY:

CALORIC INTAKE GOAL

BREAKFAST	CALORIES	FROM FAT
MEAL TOTAL:		

LUNCH	CALORIES	FROM FAT
MEAL TOTAL:		

DINNER	CALORIES	FROM FAT
MEAL TOTAL:		

SNACKS/DESSERTS	CALORIES	FROM FAT
TOTAL:		

EXERCISE	CALORIES BURNED
TOTAL CALORIES BURNED:	

CALORIE TOTALS

INTAKE	FROM FAT	BURNED	ADJUSTED

NOTES

WEEK NINE

STARTING STATS

DATE:	WEIGHT:
WAIST:	HIPS:
CHEST:	THIGHS:
CALVES:	ARMS:

NOTES/JOURNAL/GOALS

_____

_____

_____

_____

_____

_____

_____

_____

_____

_____

_____

_____

_____

_____

SUNDAY:

CALORIC INTAKE GOAL

BREAKFAST	CALORIES	FROM FAT
MEAL TOTAL:		

LUNCH	CALORIES	FROM FAT
MEAL TOTAL:		

DINNER	CALORIES	FROM FAT
MEAL TOTAL:		

SNACKS/DESSERTS	CALORIES	FROM FAT
TOTAL:		

EXERCISE	CALORIES BURNED
TOTAL CALORIES BURNED:	

CALORIE TOTALS

INTAKE	FROM FAT	BURNED	ADJUSTED

NOTES

131

MONDAY:

CALORIC INTAKE GOAL

BREAKFAST	CALORIES	FROM FAT
MEAL TOTAL:		

LUNCH	CALORIES	FROM FAT
MEAL TOTAL:		

DINNER	CALORIES	FROM FAT
MEAL TOTAL:		

132

SNACKS/DESSERTS	CALORIES	FROM FAT
TOTAL:		

EXERCISE	CALORIES BURNED
TOTAL CALORIES BURNED:	

CALORIE TOTALS

INTAKE	FROM FAT	BURNED	ADJUSTED

NOTES

TUESDAY:

CALORIC INTAKE GOAL

BREAKFAST	CALORIES	FROM FAT
MEAL TOTAL:		

LUNCH	CALORIES	FROM FAT
MEAL TOTAL:		

DINNER	CALORIES	FROM FAT
MEAL TOTAL:		

134

SNACKS/DESSERTS	CALORIES	FROM FAT
TOTAL:		

EXERCISE	CALORIES BURNED
TOTAL CALORIES BURNED:	

CALORIE TOTALS

INTAKE	FROM FAT	BURNED	ADJUSTED

NOTES

WEDNESDAY:

CALORIC INTAKE GOAL

BREAKFAST	CALORIES	FROM FAT
MEAL TOTAL:		

LUNCH	CALORIES	FROM FAT
MEAL TOTAL:		

DINNER	CALORIES	FROM FAT
MEAL TOTAL:		

SNACKS/DESSERTS	CALORIES	FROM FAT
TOTAL:		

EXERCISE	CALORIES BURNED
TOTAL CALORIES BURNED:	

CALORIE TOTALS

INTAKE	FROM FAT	BURNED	ADJUSTED

NOTES

137

THURSDAY:

CALORIC INTAKE GOAL

BREAKFAST	CALORIES	FROM FAT
MEAL TOTAL:		

LUNCH	CALORIES	FROM FAT
MEAL TOTAL:		

DINNER	CALORIES	FROM FAT
MEAL TOTAL:		

138

SNACKS/DESSERTS	CALORIES	FROM FAT
TOTAL:		

EXERCISE	CALORIES BURNED
TOTAL CALORIES BURNED:	

CALORIE TOTALS

INTAKE	FROM FAT	BURNED	ADJUSTED

NOTES

FRIDAY:

CALORIC INTAKE GOAL

BREAKFAST

	CALORIES	FROM FAT
MEAL TOTAL:		

LUNCH

	CALORIES	FROM FAT
MEAL TOTAL:		

DINNER

	CALORIES	FROM FAT
MEAL TOTAL:		

SNACKS/DESSERTS	CALORIES	FROM FAT
TOTAL:		

EXERCISE	CALORIES BURNED
TOTAL CALORIES BURNED:	

CALORIE TOTALS

INTAKE	FROM FAT	BURNED	ADJUSTED

NOTES

141

SATURDAY:

CALORIC INTAKE GOAL

BREAKFAST	CALORIES	FROM FAT
MEAL TOTAL:		

LUNCH	CALORIES	FROM FAT
MEAL TOTAL:		

DINNER	CALORIES	FROM FAT
MEAL TOTAL:		

SNACKS/DESSERTS	CALORIES	FROM FAT
TOTAL:		

EXERCISE	CALORIES BURNED
TOTAL CALORIES BURNED:	

CALORIE TOTALS

INTAKE	FROM FAT	BURNED	ADJUSTED

NOTES

143

WEEK TEN

STARTING STATS

DATE: _____   WEIGHT: _____

WAIST: _____   HIPS: _____

CHEST: _____   THIGHS: _____

CALVES: _____   ARMS: _____

_____   _____

NOTES/JOURNAL/GOALS

_____

_____

_____

_____

_____

_____

_____

_____

_____

_____

_____

_____

SUNDAY:

CALORIC INTAKE GOAL

BREAKFAST	CALORIES	FROM FAT
MEAL TOTAL:		

LUNCH	CALORIES	FROM FAT
MEAL TOTAL:		

DINNER	CALORIES	FROM FAT
MEAL TOTAL:		

146

SNACKS/DESSERTS	CALORIES	FROM FAT
TOTAL:		

EXERCISE	CALORIES BURNED
TOTAL CALORIES BURNED:	

CALORIE TOTALS

INTAKE	FROM FAT	BURNED	ADJUSTED

NOTES

MONDAY:

CALORIC INTAKE GOAL

BREAKFAST	CALORIES	FROM FAT
MEAL TOTAL:		

LUNCH	CALORIES	FROM FAT
MEAL TOTAL:		

DINNER	CALORIES	FROM FAT
MEAL TOTAL:		

SNACKS/DESSERTS	CALORIES	FROM FAT
TOTAL:		

EXERCISE	CALORIES BURNED
TOTAL CALORIES BURNED:	

CALORIE TOTALS

INTAKE	FROM FAT	BURNED	ADJUSTED

NOTES

TUESDAY:

CALORIC INTAKE GOAL

BREAKFAST	CALORIES	FROM FAT
MEAL TOTAL:		

LUNCH	CALORIES	FROM FAT
MEAL TOTAL:		

DINNER	CALORIES	FROM FAT
MEAL TOTAL:		

SNACKS/DESSERTS	CALORIES	FROM FAT
TOTAL:		

EXERCISE	CALORIES BURNED
TOTAL CALORIES BURNED:	

CALORIE TOTALS

INTAKE	FROM FAT	BURNED	ADJUSTED

NOTES

WEDNESDAY:

CALORIC INTAKE GOAL

BREAKFAST	CALORIES	FROM FAT
MEAL TOTAL:		

LUNCH	CALORIES	FROM FAT
MEAL TOTAL:		

DINNER	CALORIES	FROM FAT
MEAL TOTAL:		

SNACKS/DESSERTS	CALORIES	FROM FAT
TOTAL:		

EXERCISE	CALORIES BURNED
TOTAL CALORIES BURNED:	

CALORIE TOTALS

INTAKE	FROM FAT	BURNED	ADJUSTED

NOTES

153

THURSDAY:

CALORIC INTAKE GOAL

BREAKFAST	CALORIES	FROM FAT
MEAL TOTAL:		

LUNCH	CALORIES	FROM FAT
MEAL TOTAL:		

DINNER	CALORIES	FROM FAT
MEAL TOTAL:		

154

SNACKS/DESSERTS	CALORIES	FROM FAT
TOTAL:		

EXERCISE	CALORIES BURNED
TOTAL CALORIES BURNED:	

CALORIE TOTALS

INTAKE	FROM FAT	BURNED	ADJUSTED

NOTES

155

FRIDAY:

CALORIC INTAKE GOAL

BREAKFAST

	CALORIES	FROM FAT
MEAL TOTAL:		

LUNCH

	CALORIES	FROM FAT
MEAL TOTAL:		

DINNER

	CALORIES	FROM FAT
MEAL TOTAL:		

SNACKS/DESSERTS	CALORIES	FROM FAT
TOTAL:		

EXERCISE	CALORIES BURNED
TOTAL CALORIES BURNED:	

CALORIE TOTALS

INTAKE	FROM FAT	BURNED	ADJUSTED

NOTES

SATURDAY:

CALORIC INTAKE GOAL

BREAKFAST	CALORIES	FROM FAT
MEAL TOTAL:		

LUNCH	CALORIES	FROM FAT
MEAL TOTAL:		

DINNER	CALORIES	FROM FAT
MEAL TOTAL:		

158

SNACKS/DESSERTS	CALORIES	FROM FAT
TOTAL:		

EXERCISE	CALORIES BURNED
TOTAL CALORIES BURNED:	

CALORIE TOTALS

INTAKE	FROM FAT	BURNED	ADJUSTED

NOTES

WEEK ELEVEN

STARTING STATS

DATE:	WEIGHT:
WAIST:	HIPS:
CHEST:	THIGHS:
CALVES:	ARMS:

NOTES/JOURNAL/GOALS

SUNDAY:

CALORIC INTAKE GOAL

BREAKFAST	CALORIES	FROM FAT
MEAL TOTAL:		

LUNCH	CALORIES	FROM FAT
MEAL TOTAL:		

DINNER	CALORIES	FROM FAT
MEAL TOTAL:		

162

SNACKS/DESSERTS	CALORIES	FROM FAT
TOTAL:		

EXERCISE	CALORIES BURNED
TOTAL CALORIES BURNED:	

CALORIE TOTALS

INTAKE	FROM FAT	BURNED	ADJUSTED

NOTES

MONDAY:

CALORIC INTAKE GOAL

BREAKFAST	CALORIES	FROM FAT
MEAL TOTAL:		

LUNCH	CALORIES	FROM FAT
MEAL TOTAL:		

DINNER	CALORIES	FROM FAT
MEAL TOTAL:		

SNACKS/DESSERTS

	CALORIES	FROM FAT
TOTAL:		

EXERCISE

	CALORIES BURNED
TOTAL CALORIES BURNED:	

CALORIE TOTALS

INTAKE	FROM FAT	BURNED	ADJUSTED

NOTES

TUESDAY:

CALORIC INTAKE GOAL

BREAKFAST	CALORIES	FROM FAT
MEAL TOTAL:		

LUNCH	CALORIES	FROM FAT
MEAL TOTAL:		

DINNER	CALORIES	FROM FAT
MEAL TOTAL:		

166

SNACKS/DESSERTS	CALORIES	FROM FAT
TOTAL:		

EXERCISE	CALORIES BURNED
TOTAL CALORIES BURNED:	

CALORIE TOTALS

INTAKE	FROM FAT	BURNED	ADJUSTED

NOTES

WEDNESDAY:

CALORIC INTAKE GOAL

BREAKFAST	CALORIES	FROM FAT
MEAL TOTAL:		

LUNCH	CALORIES	FROM FAT
MEAL TOTAL:		

DINNER	CALORIES	FROM FAT
MEAL TOTAL:		

SNACKS/DESSERTS	CALORIES	FROM FAT
TOTAL:		

EXERCISE	CALORIES BURNED
TOTAL CALORIES BURNED:	

CALORIE TOTALS

INTAKE	FROM FAT	BURNED	ADJUSTED

NOTES

THURSDAY:

CALORIC INTAKE GOAL

BREAKFAST	CALORIES	FROM FAT
MEAL TOTAL:		

LUNCH	CALORIES	FROM FAT
MEAL TOTAL:		

DINNER	CALORIES	FROM FAT
MEAL TOTAL:		

170

SNACKS/DESSERTS	CALORIES	FROM FAT
TOTAL:		

EXERCISE	CALORIES BURNED
TOTAL CALORIES BURNED:	

CALORIE TOTALS

INTAKE	FROM FAT	BURNED	ADJUSTED

NOTES

FRIDAY:

CALORIC INTAKE GOAL

BREAKFAST	CALORIES	FROM FAT
MEAL TOTAL:		

LUNCH	CALORIES	FROM FAT
MEAL TOTAL:		

DINNER	CALORIES	FROM FAT
MEAL TOTAL:		

172

SNACKS/DESSERTS	CALORIES	FROM FAT
TOTAL:		

EXERCISE	CALORIES BURNED
TOTAL CALORIES BURNED:	

CALORIE TOTALS

INTAKE	FROM FAT	BURNED	ADJUSTED

NOTES

173

SATURDAY:

BREAKFAST	CALORIES	FROM FAT
MEAL TOTAL:		

LUNCH	CALORIES	FROM FAT
MEAL TOTAL:		

DINNER	CALORIES	FROM FAT
MEAL TOTAL:		

SNACKS/DESSERTS	CALORIES	FROM FAT
TOTAL:		

EXERCISE	CALORIES BURNED
TOTAL CALORIES BURNED:	

CALORIE TOTALS

INTAKE	FROM FAT	BURNED	ADJUSTED

NOTES

WEEK TWELVE

STARTING STATS

DATE:	WEIGHT:
WAIST:	HIPS:
CHEST:	THIGHS:
CALVES:	ARMS:

NOTES/JOURNAL/GOALS

SUNDAY:

CALORIC INTAKE GOAL

BREAKFAST	CALORIES	FROM FAT
MEAL TOTAL:		

LUNCH	CALORIES	FROM FAT
MEAL TOTAL:		

DINNER	CALORIES	FROM FAT
MEAL TOTAL:		

SNACKS/DESSERTS	CALORIES	FROM FAT
TOTAL:		

EXERCISE	CALORIES BURNED
TOTAL CALORIES BURNED:	

CALORIE TOTALS

INTAKE	FROM FAT	BURNED	ADJUSTED

NOTES

MONDAY:

CALORIC INTAKE GOAL

BREAKFAST	CALORIES	FROM FAT
MEAL TOTAL:		

LUNCH	CALORIES	FROM FAT
MEAL TOTAL:		

DINNER	CALORIES	FROM FAT
MEAL TOTAL:		

SNACKS/DESSERTS	CALORIES	FROM FAT
TOTAL:		

EXERCISE	CALORIES BURNED
TOTAL CALORIES BURNED:	

CALORIE TOTALS

INTAKE	FROM FAT	BURNED	ADJUSTED

NOTES

TUESDAY:

CALORIC INTAKE GOAL

BREAKFAST	CALORIES	FROM FAT
MEAL TOTAL:		

LUNCH	CALORIES	FROM FAT
MEAL TOTAL:		

DINNER	CALORIES	FROM FAT
MEAL TOTAL:		

SNACKS/DESSERTS	CALORIES	FROM FAT
TOTAL:		

EXERCISE	CALORIES BURNED
TOTAL CALORIES BURNED:	

CALORIE TOTALS

INTAKE	FROM FAT	BURNED	ADJUSTED

NOTES

WEDNESDAY:

CALORIC INTAKE GOAL

BREAKFAST

	CALORIES	FROM FAT
MEAL TOTAL:		

LUNCH

	CALORIES	FROM FAT
MEAL TOTAL:		

DINNER

	CALORIES	FROM FAT
MEAL TOTAL:		

SNACKS/DESSERTS	CALORIES	FROM FAT
TOTAL:		

EXERCISE	CALORIES BURNED
TOTAL CALORIES BURNED:	

CALORIE TOTALS

INTAKE	FROM FAT	BURNED	ADJUSTED

NOTES

185

THURSDAY:

CALORIC INTAKE GOAL

BREAKFAST

	CALORIES	FROM FAT
MEAL TOTAL:		

LUNCH

	CALORIES	FROM FAT
MEAL TOTAL:		

DINNER

	CALORIES	FROM FAT
MEAL TOTAL:		

SNACKS/DESSERTS	CALORIES	FROM FAT
TOTAL:		

EXERCISE	CALORIES BURNED
TOTAL CALORIES BURNED:	

CALORIE TOTALS

INTAKE	FROM FAT	BURNED	ADJUSTED

NOTES

_____

_____

_____

_____

FRIDAY:

CALORIC INTAKE GOAL

BREAKFAST	CALORIES	FROM FAT
MEAL TOTAL:		

LUNCH	CALORIES	FROM FAT
MEAL TOTAL:		

DINNER	CALORIES	FROM FAT
MEAL TOTAL:		

SNACKS/DESSERTS	CALORIES	FROM FAT
TOTAL:		

EXERCISE	CALORIES BURNED
TOTAL CALORIES BURNED:	

CALORIE TOTALS

INTAKE	FROM FAT	BURNED	ADJUSTED

NOTES

SATURDAY:

CALORIC INTAKE GOAL

BREAKFAST	CALORIES	FROM FAT
MEAL TOTAL:		

LUNCH	CALORIES	FROM FAT
MEAL TOTAL:		

DINNER	CALORIES	FROM FAT
MEAL TOTAL:		

SNACKS/DESSERTS	CALORIES	FROM FAT
TOTAL:		

EXERCISE	CALORIES BURNED
TOTAL CALORIES BURNED:	

CALORIE TOTALS

INTAKE	FROM FAT	BURNED	ADJUSTED

NOTES

WEEK THIRTEEN

STARTING STATS

DATE:	WEIGHT:
WAIST:	HIPS:
CHEST:	THIGHS:
CALVES:	ARMS:

NOTES/JOURNAL/GOALS

SUNDAY:

CALORIC INTAKE GOAL

BREAKFAST	CALORIES	FROM FAT
MEAL TOTAL:		

LUNCH	CALORIES	FROM FAT
MEAL TOTAL:		

DINNER	CALORIES	FROM FAT
MEAL TOTAL:		

SNACKS/DESSERTS	CALORIES	FROM FAT
TOTAL:		

EXERCISE	CALORIES BURNED
TOTAL CALORIES BURNED:	

CALORIE TOTALS

INTAKE	FROM FAT	BURNED	ADJUSTED

NOTES

MONDAY:

CALORIC INTAKE GOAL

BREAKFAST	CALORIES	FROM FAT
MEAL TOTAL:		

LUNCH	CALORIES	FROM FAT
MEAL TOTAL:		

DINNER	CALORIES	FROM FAT
MEAL TOTAL:		

196

SNACKS/DESSERTS	CALORIES	FROM FAT
TOTAL:		

EXERCISE	CALORIES BURNED
TOTAL CALORIES BURNED:	

CALORIE TOTALS

INTAKE	FROM FAT	BURNED	ADJUSTED

NOTES

197

TUESDAY:

CALORIC INTAKE GOAL

BREAKFAST	CALORIES	FROM FAT
MEAL TOTAL:		

LUNCH	CALORIES	FROM FAT
MEAL TOTAL:		

DINNER	CALORIES	FROM FAT
MEAL TOTAL:		

SNACKS/DESSERTS	CALORIES	FROM FAT
TOTAL:		

EXERCISE	CALORIES BURNED
TOTAL CALORIES BURNED:	

CALORIE TOTALS

INTAKE	FROM FAT	BURNED	ADJUSTED

NOTES

199

WEDNESDAY:

CALORIC INTAKE GOAL

BREAKFAST	CALORIES	FROM FAT
MEAL TOTAL:		

LUNCH	CALORIES	FROM FAT
MEAL TOTAL:		

DINNER	CALORIES	FROM FAT
MEAL TOTAL:		

SNACKS/DESSERTS	CALORIES	FROM FAT
TOTAL:		

EXERCISE	CALORIES BURNED
TOTAL CALORIES BURNED:	

CALORIE TOTALS

INTAKE	FROM FAT	BURNED	ADJUSTED

NOTES

THURSDAY:

CALORIC INTAKE GOAL

BREAKFAST	CALORIES	FROM FAT
MEAL TOTAL:		

LUNCH	CALORIES	FROM FAT
MEAL TOTAL:		

DINNER	CALORIES	FROM FAT
MEAL TOTAL:		

SNACKS/DESSERTS	CALORIES	FROM FAT
TOTAL:		

EXERCISE	CALORIES BURNED
TOTAL CALORIES BURNED:	

CALORIE TOTALS

INTAKE	FROM FAT	BURNED	ADJUSTED

NOTES

203

FRIDAY:

CALORIC INTAKE GOAL

BREAKFAST

	CALORIES	FROM FAT
MEAL TOTAL:		

LUNCH

	CALORIES	FROM FAT
MEAL TOTAL:		

DINNER

	CALORIES	FROM FAT
MEAL TOTAL:		

SNACKS/DESSERTS	CALORIES	FROM FAT
TOTAL:		

EXERCISE	CALORIES BURNED
TOTAL CALORIES BURNED:	

CALORIE TOTALS

INTAKE	FROM FAT	BURNED	ADJUSTED

NOTES

SATURDAY:

CALORIC INTAKE GOAL

BREAKFAST	CALORIES	FROM FAT
MEAL TOTAL:		

LUNCH	CALORIES	FROM FAT
MEAL TOTAL:		

DINNER	CALORIES	FROM FAT
MEAL TOTAL:		

SNACKS/DESSERTS	CALORIES	FROM FAT
TOTAL:		

EXERCISE	CALORIES BURNED
TOTAL CALORIES BURNED:	

CALORIE TOTALS

INTAKE	FROM FAT	BURNED	ADJUSTED

NOTES

WEEK FOURTEEN

STARTING STATS

DATE:	WEIGHT:
WAIST:	HIPS:
CHEST:	THIGHS:
CALVES:	ARMS:

NOTES/JOURNAL/GOALS

SUNDAY:

CALORIC INTAKE GOAL

BREAKFAST	CALORIES	FROM FAT
MEAL TOTAL:		

LUNCH	CALORIES	FROM FAT
MEAL TOTAL:		

DINNER	CALORIES	FROM FAT
MEAL TOTAL:		

SNACKS/DESSERTS	CALORIES	FROM FAT
TOTAL:		

EXERCISE	CALORIES BURNED
TOTAL CALORIES BURNED:	

CALORIE TOTALS

INTAKE	FROM FAT	BURNED	ADJUSTED

NOTES

MONDAY:

CALORIC INTAKE GOAL

BREAKFAST	CALORIES	FROM FAT
MEAL TOTAL:		

LUNCH	CALORIES	FROM FAT
MEAL TOTAL:		

DINNER	CALORIES	FROM FAT
MEAL TOTAL:		

SNACKS/DESSERTS	CALORIES	FROM FAT
TOTAL:		

EXERCISE	CALORIES BURNED
TOTAL CALORIES BURNED:	

CALORIE TOTALS

INTAKE	FROM FAT	BURNED	ADJUSTED

NOTES

TUESDAY:

CALORIC INTAKE GOAL

BREAKFAST	CALORIES	FROM FAT
MEAL TOTAL:		

LUNCH	CALORIES	FROM FAT
MEAL TOTAL:		

DINNER	CALORIES	FROM FAT
MEAL TOTAL:		

SNACKS/DESSERTS

	CALORIES	FROM FAT
TOTAL:		

EXERCISE

	CALORIES BURNED
TOTAL CALORIES BURNED:	

CALORIE TOTALS

INTAKE	FROM FAT	BURNED	ADJUSTED

NOTES

215

WEDNESDAY:

CALORIC INTAKE GOAL

BREAKFAST	CALORIES	FROM FAT
MEAL TOTAL:		

LUNCH	CALORIES	FROM FAT
MEAL TOTAL:		

DINNER	CALORIES	FROM FAT
MEAL TOTAL:		

SNACKS/DESSERTS	CALORIES	FROM FAT
TOTAL:		

EXERCISE	CALORIES BURNED
TOTAL CALORIES BURNED:	

CALORIE TOTALS

INTAKE	FROM FAT	BURNED	ADJUSTED

NOTES

THURSDAY:

CALORIC INTAKE GOAL

BREAKFAST	CALORIES	FROM FAT
MEAL TOTAL:		

LUNCH	CALORIES	FROM FAT
MEAL TOTAL:		

DINNER	CALORIES	FROM FAT
MEAL TOTAL:		

SNACKS/DESSERTS	CALORIES	FROM FAT
TOTAL:		

EXERCISE	CALORIES BURNED
TOTAL CALORIES BURNED:	

CALORIE TOTALS

INTAKE	FROM FAT	BURNED	ADJUSTED

NOTES

FRIDAY:

CALORIC INTAKE GOAL

BREAKFAST	CALORIES	FROM FAT
MEAL TOTAL:		

LUNCH	CALORIES	FROM FAT
MEAL TOTAL:		

DINNER	CALORIES	FROM FAT
MEAL TOTAL:		

SNACKS/DESSERTS	CALORIES	FROM FAT
TOTAL:		

EXERCISE	CALORIES BURNED
TOTAL CALORIES BURNED:	

CALORIE TOTALS

INTAKE	FROM FAT	BURNED	ADJUSTED

NOTES

SATURDAY:

CALORIC INTAKE GOAL

BREAKFAST

	CALORIES	FROM FAT
MEAL TOTAL:		

LUNCH

	CALORIES	FROM FAT
MEAL TOTAL:		

DINNER

	CALORIES	FROM FAT
MEAL TOTAL:		

SNACKS/DESSERTS	CALORIES	FROM FAT
TOTAL:		

EXERCISE	CALORIES BURNED
TOTAL CALORIES BURNED:	

CALORIE TOTALS

INTAKE	FROM FAT	BURNED	ADJUSTED

NOTES

WEEK FIFTEEN

STARTING STATS

DATE:	WEIGHT:
WAIST:	HIPS:
CHEST:	THIGHS:
CALVES:	ARMS:

NOTES/JOURNAL/GOALS

SUNDAY:

CALORIC INTAKE GOAL

BREAKFAST	CALORIES	FROM FAT
MEAL TOTAL:		

LUNCH	CALORIES	FROM FAT
MEAL TOTAL:		

DINNER	CALORIES	FROM FAT
MEAL TOTAL:		

SNACKS/DESSERTS	CALORIES	FROM FAT
TOTAL:		

EXERCISE	CALORIES BURNED
TOTAL CALORIES BURNED:	

CALORIE TOTALS

INTAKE	FROM FAT	BURNED	ADJUSTED

NOTES

MONDAY:

CALORIC INTAKE GOAL

BREAKFAST	CALORIES	FROM FAT
MEAL TOTAL:		

LUNCH	CALORIES	FROM FAT
MEAL TOTAL:		

DINNER	CALORIES	FROM FAT
MEAL TOTAL:		

SNACKS/DESSERTS	CALORIES	FROM FAT
TOTAL:		

EXERCISE	CALORIES BURNED
TOTAL CALORIES BURNED:	

CALORIE TOTALS

INTAKE	FROM FAT	BURNED	ADJUSTED

NOTES

TUESDAY:

CALORIC INTAKE GOAL

BREAKFAST	CALORIES	FROM FAT
MEAL TOTAL:		

LUNCH	CALORIES	FROM FAT
MEAL TOTAL:		

DINNER	CALORIES	FROM FAT
MEAL TOTAL:		

SNACKS/DESSERTS	CALORIES	FROM FAT
TOTAL:		

EXERCISE	CALORIES BURNED
TOTAL CALORIES BURNED:	

CALORIE TOTALS

INTAKE	FROM FAT	BURNED	ADJUSTED

NOTES

WEDNESDAY:

CALORIC INTAKE GOAL

BREAKFAST	CALORIES	FROM FAT
MEAL TOTAL:		

LUNCH	CALORIES	FROM FAT
MEAL TOTAL:		

DINNER	CALORIES	FROM FAT
MEAL TOTAL:		

SNACKS/DESSERTS	CALORIES	FROM FAT
TOTAL:		

EXERCISE	CALORIES BURNED
TOTAL CALORIES BURNED:	

CALORIE TOTALS

INTAKE	FROM FAT	BURNED	ADJUSTED

NOTES

THURSDAY:

CALORIC INTAKE GOAL

BREAKFAST	CALORIES	FROM FAT
MEAL TOTAL:		

LUNCH	CALORIES	FROM FAT
MEAL TOTAL:		

DINNER	CALORIES	FROM FAT
MEAL TOTAL:		

SNACKS/DESSERTS	CALORIES	FROM FAT
TOTAL:		

EXERCISE	CALORIES BURNED
TOTAL CALORIES BURNED:	

CALORIE TOTALS

INTAKE	FROM FAT	BURNED	ADJUSTED

NOTES

FRIDAY:

CALORIC INTAKE GOAL

BREAKFAST	CALORIES	FROM FAT
MEAL TOTAL:		

LUNCH	CALORIES	FROM FAT
MEAL TOTAL:		

DINNER	CALORIES	FROM FAT
MEAL TOTAL:		

SNACKS/DESSERTS	CALORIES	FROM FAT
TOTAL:		

EXERCISE	CALORIES BURNED
TOTAL CALORIES BURNED:	

CALORIE TOTALS

INTAKE	FROM FAT	BURNED	ADJUSTED

NOTES

SATURDAY:

CALORIC INTAKE GOAL

BREAKFAST	CALORIES	FROM FAT
MEAL TOTAL:		

LUNCH	CALORIES	FROM FAT
MEAL TOTAL:		

DINNER	CALORIES	FROM FAT
MEAL TOTAL:		

238

SNACKS/DESSERTS	CALORIES	FROM FAT
TOTAL:		

EXERCISE	CALORIES BURNED
TOTAL CALORIES BURNED:	

CALORIE TOTALS

INTAKE	FROM FAT	BURNED	ADJUSTED

NOTES

WEEK SIXTEEN

STARTING STATS

DATE:	WEIGHT:
WAIST:	HIPS:
CHEST:	THIGHS:
CALVES:	ARMS:

NOTES/JOURNAL/GOALS

SUNDAY:

CALORIC INTAKE GOAL

BREAKFAST	CALORIES	FROM FAT
MEAL TOTAL:		

LUNCH	CALORIES	FROM FAT
MEAL TOTAL:		

DINNER	CALORIES	FROM FAT
MEAL TOTAL:		

SNACKS/DESSERTS	CALORIES	FROM FAT
TOTAL:		

EXERCISE	CALORIES BURNED
TOTAL CALORIES BURNED:	

CALORIE TOTALS

INTAKE	FROM FAT	BURNED	ADJUSTED

NOTES

_____

_____

_____

_____

MONDAY:

CALORIC INTAKE GOAL

BREAKFAST	CALORIES	FROM FAT
MEAL TOTAL:		

LUNCH	CALORIES	FROM FAT
MEAL TOTAL:		

DINNER	CALORIES	FROM FAT
MEAL TOTAL:		

SNACKS/DESSERTS	CALORIES	FROM FAT
TOTAL:		

EXERCISE	CALORIES BURNED
TOTAL CALORIES BURNED:	

CALORIE TOTALS

INTAKE	FROM FAT	BURNED	ADJUSTED

NOTES

245

TUESDAY:

CALORIC INTAKE GOAL

BREAKFAST	CALORIES	FROM FAT
MEAL TOTAL:		

LUNCH	CALORIES	FROM FAT
MEAL TOTAL:		

DINNER	CALORIES	FROM FAT
MEAL TOTAL:		

SNACKS/DESSERTS	CALORIES	FROM FAT
TOTAL:		

EXERCISE	CALORIES BURNED
TOTAL CALORIES BURNED:	

CALORIE TOTALS

INTAKE	FROM FAT	BURNED	ADJUSTED

NOTES

WEDNESDAY:

CALORIC INTAKE GOAL

BREAKFAST	CALORIES	FROM FAT
MEAL TOTAL:		

LUNCH	CALORIES	FROM FAT
MEAL TOTAL:		

DINNER	CALORIES	FROM FAT
MEAL TOTAL:		

SNACKS/DESSERTS	CALORIES	FROM FAT
TOTAL:		

EXERCISE	CALORIES BURNED
TOTAL CALORIES BURNED:	

CALORIE TOTALS

INTAKE	FROM FAT	BURNED	ADJUSTED

NOTES

THURSDAY:

CALORIC INTAKE GOAL

BREAKFAST	CALORIES	FROM FAT
MEAL TOTAL:		

LUNCH	CALORIES	FROM FAT
MEAL TOTAL:		

DINNER	CALORIES	FROM FAT
MEAL TOTAL:		

SNACKS/DESSERTS	CALORIES	FROM FAT
TOTAL:		

EXERCISE	CALORIES BURNED
TOTAL CALORIES BURNED:	

CALORIE TOTALS

INTAKE	FROM FAT	BURNED	ADJUSTED

NOTES

FRIDAY:

BREAKFAST	CALORIES	FROM FAT
MEAL TOTAL:		

LUNCH	CALORIES	FROM FAT
MEAL TOTAL:		

DINNER	CALORIES	FROM FAT
MEAL TOTAL:		

252

SNACKS/DESSERTS	CALORIES	FROM FAT
TOTAL:		

EXERCISE	CALORIES BURNED
TOTAL CALORIES BURNED:	

CALORIE TOTALS

INTAKE	FROM FAT	BURNED	ADJUSTED

NOTES

SATURDAY:

CALORIC INTAKE GOAL

BREAKFAST	CALORIES	FROM FAT
MEAL TOTAL:		

LUNCH	CALORIES	FROM FAT
MEAL TOTAL:		

DINNER	CALORIES	FROM FAT
MEAL TOTAL:		

SNACKS/DESSERTS	CALORIES	FROM FAT
TOTAL:		

EXERCISE	CALORIES BURNED
TOTAL CALORIES BURNED:	

CALORIE TOTALS

INTAKE	FROM FAT	BURNED	ADJUSTED

NOTES

NOTES/JOURNAL

Printed in the United States
76724LV00002B/171

9 780976 807650